# A CHRISTIAN PERSPECTIVE
## *on*
# CHINESE MEDICINE

*Pak-Wah Lai, PhD*

Illustrated by Wendy Wong

GRACEWORKS

*For Rina, Chin-Loon and Chor-Tiang*

*A Christian Perspective on Chinese Medicine*

Copyright © 2021 Lai Pak-Wah

All rights reserved. No part of this publication may be reproduced, stored in a retrieval system, or transmitted, in any form or by any means, electronic, mechanical, photocopying, recording or otherwise, without the prior written permission of the authors, except in the case of brief quotations embodied in critical articles and reviews.

Published by Graceworks Private Limited
22 Sin Ming Lane
#04-76 Midview City
Singapore 573969
Tel: 67523403
Email: enquiries@graceworks.com.sg
Website: www.graceworks.com.sg

All Scripture quotations, unless otherwise noted, are taken from *The Holy Bible, New International Version*®. NIV®. Copyright © 1973, 1978, 1984, 2011 by International Bible Society. Used by permission of Zondervan. All rights reserved.

Illustrations by Wendy Wong
Body text typeset in Arno Pro

ISBN: 978-981-14-8941-9

1 2 3 4 5 6 7 8 9 10 · 27 26 25 24 23 22 21

I found *A Christian Perspective on Chinese Medicine* to be refreshingly simple, helpful and clear about a daunting topic plagued by ignorance, fear and instinctive reactions. This booklet provides an overview of the key areas of consideration, making it suitable as a standalone resource for rapid appreciation of the subject matter and provides the impetus for further reading. The approach outlined is accessible and provides a framework for deeper theological reflection and practice. I highly commend this booklet for your prayerful reading.

*~ Dr Ng Liang Wei, Pastor, Mt Carmel Bible Presbyterian Church*

Apart from Western medicine that dominates our healthcare system, can one turn to alternative medicine? In this highly engaging and readable booklet, Dr Lai provides a biblical and theological framework for understanding medicine, and carefully evaluates Traditional Chinese Medicine which has often been viewed suspiciously by Asian Christians. This is one of the very rare resources available that deals with this subject sensitively and biblically.

*~ Rev Dr Lim Kar Yong, Seminari Theologi Malaysia*

Having grown up a Christian in an English congregation, I was warned against pursuing Chinese medicine. A prayer warrior in church even came to share her utmost concern about other spiritual forces behind its practices. This book helpfully dissects the history and philosophy behind both Western and Chinese medical traditions. It not only provides a systematic understanding about how Chinese medicine is shaped by the immense complexities of Chinese culture, but also covers the legitimacy of Chinese medicine from a theology perspective. All while brilliantly leading us back to the center of healing, i.e.: our Lord Jesus Christ, the ultimate healer!

*~ Joanna Liew, TCM Physician and Asst Director, Healthcare Division, Perennial Holdings Private Limited*

In *A Christian Perspective on Chinese Medicine*, Dr Lai offers a clear and informative overview of Western and Chinese medicine, expounding on their origins, limits and differences in a systematic manner. In his typical engaging manner, he fills the gaps in the readers' understanding, and addresses the concerns of the Christian community with regards to Chinese medicine. An interesting and easy-to-read book for those who are keen to know more about Chinese medicine.

> *~ Ho Shen Yong, Principal Lecturer, Physics and Applied Physics;*
> *Associate Dean (Academic), College of Science, NTU*

Traditional Chinese Medicine is intimately related to Chinese history and culture. As such, it is a topic that Christians in Asia need to take seriously. Recognising the value and limits of Chinese medicine, Dr Lai's treatment of the subject is competent, nuanced, balanced and theologically informed. Besides deepening our understanding of the subject, it places in the hands of Christian readers significant resources by which to build bridges with our Chinese neighbours in our multi-cultural society.

> *~ Dr Edwin Tay, Principal, Trinity Theological College*

Dr Lai is not only a theologian but also someone who has done extensive research in the field of Traditional Chinese Medicine (TCM). His earnest examination of Chinese medicine from a biblical and theological perspective has helped Christians overcome their doubts and suspicions of the subject. This avoids the scenario where Christian misunderstanding about TCM causes the non-Christian Chinese to be biased against Christianity. This book is very readable and a good reference for the subject.

> *~ Rev Dr Caleb Soo, Moderator, Singapore Life Church*

Foreword **ix**

*Introduction* **01**

*Biblical and Theological Perspectives on Medicine* **07**

*Evaluating Western Medical Traditions* **19**

*Evaluating Chinese Medical Tradition* **25**

*Conclusion* **37**

Endnotes **40**

## FOREWORD

Ever since the publication of *The Dao of Healing: Christian Perspectives on Chinese Medicine* in 2018, there have been several requests for a more popular level or simpler version of the book. As a result of the numerous invitations to speak on this subject, I have since condensed my ideas for the general public. It seems a right time for me to put them into writing. Readers should note, however, that I will not be discussing the scientific legitimacy of Chinese medicine here. While it is an important subject, a proper treatment of it would require a far more extensive discussion. That will detract us from the aim of this book, which is to address the theological concerns about Chinese medicine. The scientific concerns have already been dealt with in Chapters 9 and 10 of *The Dao of Healing*. Readers are advised to consult them instead.

A book project is never a solitary endeavour. Behind a book is always the strong support of our families and friends. This is certainly the case for me. I would like to thank, first of all, my colleagues at the Biblical Graduate School of Theology (BGST) for their continual support, and the churches who invited me over the past two years. The latter, in particular, have provided me with many opportunities to develop what I shall be presenting here.

My appreciation also goes to my editor and publisher, Bernice Tan, for encouraging the publication of this booklet. Much gratitude also goes to my wife, Rina. In November 2019, I had a bad cycling accident and could not use my arms for two whole weeks. It was the crucial period when Dr Diarra Boubachar and I had to deliver two lecture series on 'Christian Perspectives on Chinese Medicine in Singapore'. Without Rina's logistics support, we would not have been able to deliver these talks successfully.

Finally, both old and new friends have helped us along the way too. Many thanks to Chai Chin-Loon and Chor-Tiang, who kindly hosted Diarra during his visits. I am grateful also for the partnership of Joanna Liew, Li Hai-Feng, David Huang and Wendy Wong. The first three are Chinese medical physicians whom I've gotten to known since the launch of *The Dao of Healing*. They have also become fellow organisers of the first Mandarin conference on 'Christian Perspectives on Chinese Medicine' in November 2019, hosted by Bukit Panjang Methodist Church. Wendy has been BGST's 'resident visual recorder' since 2019 and is a joy to work with. She is also the illustrator of the beautiful graphics in this booklet.

It is my prayer that this booklet will be a blessing for fellow Christians and provide fresh impetus for them to engage the Chinese community.

INTRODUCTION I

Whenever the name Huang Fei Hong is mentioned (黄飞鸿, 1847–1925), fans of Hong Kong movies would immediately recognise him as a grandmaster in Chinese martial arts. Huang is not just a martial arts expert, however. After a stint training sailors from the Guangzhou navy, Huang went on to set up Bao Zhi Lin (宝芝林), a medical hall, where he practised Chinese medicine for several years. This aspect of Huang's life is well expressed in Jet Li's *Huang Fei Hong* movie, where he apparently demonstrated the use of acupuncture needles before a class of Western medical doctors.

However, Chinese medicine did not originate in the Qing Dynasty. Its historical roots run much deeper and may be traced to as early as 400 BC (the Warring States era). It is for this reason that acupuncture and moxibustion were both recognised by UNESCO as forms of Intangible Cultural Heritage of Humanity in 2010.[1]

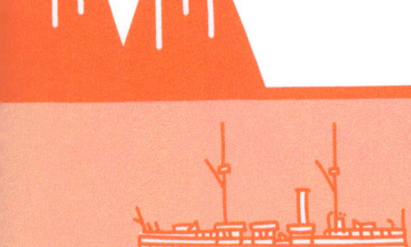

This being said, there are many Christians who are suspicious of the Chinese medical tradition and actively discourage Christians from using it, let alone practise it as Chinese medical physicians. Their concern is not just the scientific legitimacy of Chinese medicine, but whether the discipline has been tainted by Daoist roots. Some argue that Chinese medical theories (particularly the concepts of *yinyang* and *qi*) are not only unscientific and unattested to by biblical teachings, but are also hindered by Daoist philosophy. For these reasons, Christians should not consult nor practise Chinese medicine.[2]

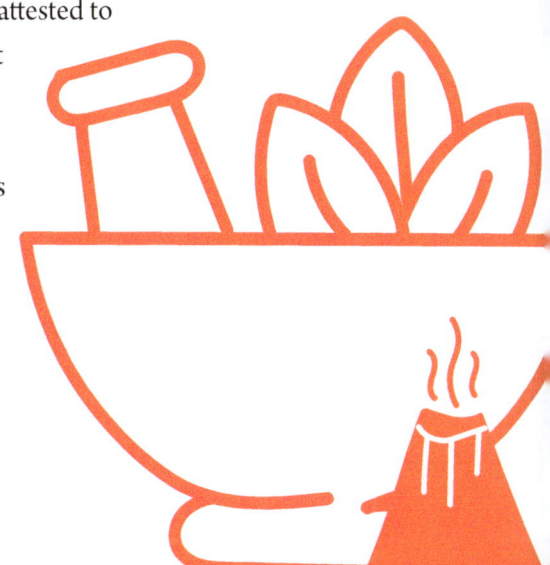

Not all Christians agree with this assessment, however. Many Chinese-speaking Christians consult Chinese medical physicians regularly. Their diet is also often informed by Chinese medical principles. And there are a growing number of Christian Chinese medicine practitioners. Some even use it as a form of medical service in their churches' outreach to their communities. Pastor Moses Pi, for example, is not only a pastor of Bethel AOG's Mandarin service but also holds a doctorate in Chinese medicine. Twice a week, he offers free Chinese medical consultations as part of the church's service to its community.[3]

Such disagreements then beg the question, "Can Christians use Chinese medicine?" It is crucial for us to answer this question carefully for the following reasons.

1. The non-Christian Chinese community often regards Christianity as a Western religion that undermines and looks down on Chinese culture, Chinese medicine being a significant aspect of it. If our dismissal or rejection of Chinese medicine is not based on robust theological and medical grounds, we alienate the non-Christian community

and create an unnecessary stumbling block to the Gospel. What is at stake, therefore, is the love of our neighbour: that we seek to understand their culture correctly, and to remove any possible opposition to the Gospel.

2. If Chinese medicine is a legitimate form of medicine, it becomes another viable therapeutic option for Christians. This can only improve the health and well-being of the Christian community.

3. Finally, a study of Chinese medicine requires us to have a better grasp of Chinese philosophy and culture. Which will be helpful when we seek to contextualise the Gospel for the Chinese.

How should we proceed then?

1. Medicine is but a means to an end — the cure or alleviation of human illness. Our study must thus begin with an exploration of how illness became prevalent and whether the use of medicine is endorsed by Scripture.

2. As we shall see, the Bible does affirm the use of medicine but does not prescribe any specific medical theories or principles. Nonetheless, we can construct a theology of medicine, which will allow us to assess the theological basis of a medical theory and its practice.

3. Having established this 'theology of medicine', we shall turn to the histories and philosophies of the Western and Chinese medical traditions, and examine how they fare against this theological benchmark.

BIBLICAL
AND
THEOLOGICAL
PERSPECTIVES
ON
MEDICINE

## Biblical Origins and Reasons for Illness

So, what does the Bible have to say about medicine in general? More importantly, how did illness and death arise in humankind?

Our study must begin with Genesis 3, where we find the serpent misleading Adam and Eve to partake of the fruit from the tree of the knowledge of good and evil. The net result is that they were banished from the Garden of Eden, condemned to suffer and eventually die. As Romans 5:12 puts it,

*Therefore, just as sin entered the world through one man, and death through sin, and in this way death came to all people, because all sinned.*

Since then, every civilisation that we know — from the Babylonians and Egyptians to the Greeks — has developed forms of medicine to treat the sick among them. When we turn to the Bible, we find instances where the use of medicine is affirmed, particularly in the New Testament. The apostle Paul hints at this when he describes Luke, his fellow evangelist, as not only his "dear friend" but also a "doctor." Later, in 1 Timothy 5:23, Paul even provides Timothy some rudimentary medical advice:

*Stop drinking only water, and use a little wine because of your stomach and your frequent illnesses.*

While most Roman cities had access to water, not all had clean, potable water (if at all!). If one had a weak stomach, he may not have been able to adapt to the local water resources. This is why Paul recommended Timothy add a little wine to his water, so as to disinfect it.

When we turn to the Christians living in the first few centuries (known otherwise as the church fathers), we find them likewise affirming medicine as a gift of God — His providential means of relieving human suffering. Nevertheless, they also recognised that medicine can never be an elixir of immortality. On the contrary, sickness and death are inevitable facts of life and will only be eradicated at the general resurrection.[4]

The fourth century is the earliest period where we find Christians discussing medical theories. Time and again, what they propound is not some form of unique Christian medical theory. Rather, it is the mainstream medicine used by everyone (Christian and non-Christian) during their day: Galenic-

Hippocratic medicine. More will be said later about this Greek medical tradition. What is noteworthy is the fact that these church fathers did spend much time discussing the different reasons for illnesses.

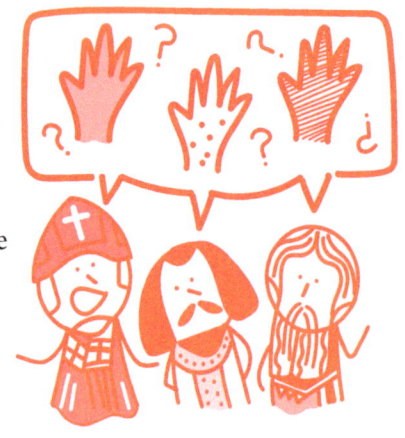

Illness, of course, will arise when one ages, and 'wear and tear' occurs. However, there are also theological reasons for sicknesses.

1. An illness can be meted out upon us **because of our sins**. This is well illustrated in Exodus 9:8–12, where we find the Egyptians inflicted with boils because the Pharaoh refused to acknowledge Yahweh as the true and living God. A similar case also occurred in 2 Kings 5:25–27, where leprosy broke out on Gehazi's skin because he was disobedient to God.

2. An illness can also come upon us, not because of any sin on our part, but **for the sake of our spiritual training and maturity**. The best example for this is Paul's thorn in the flesh in 2 Corinthians 12. Time and again, Paul pleaded with God to remove this thorn. Yet, the response he got from God was this: "My grace is sufficient for you, for my power is made perfect in weakness" (2 Cor 12:9). In

other words, God wanted to use this thorn as the means of training Paul so that the apostle may learn to minister not according to his own strength but by the grace and power of God!

3. An illness can happen as **a spiritual or religious symbol**. In Genesis 32, God wrestled with Jacob overnight before He touched and injured Jacob's hip. Henceforth, the patriarch would walk with a limp, a reminder that he once wrestled with God but survived miraculously!

4. One may suffer from an illness or disability **for the sake of God's glory**. This is certainly the case for the man born blind (John 9), whose healing was to glorify God before the Jews.

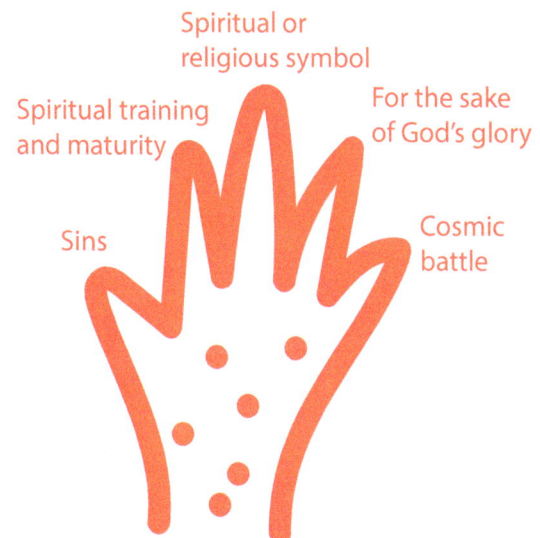

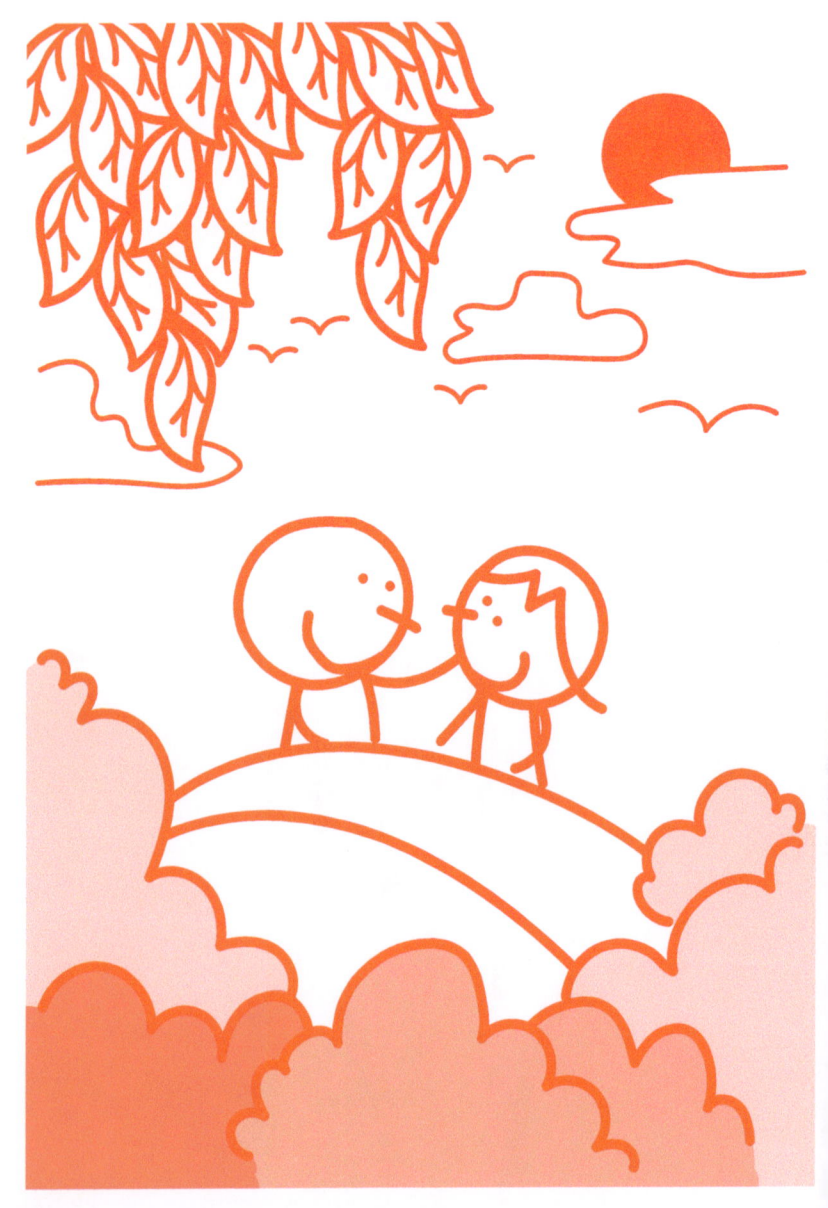

5. Our illnesses may be the **arena for a cosmic battle between God and Satan**. Such is the case for Job, whose boils were due to no sin of his, but to test and demonstrate his faith to Satan (Job 2).

## A Theology of Medicine

### *All Things were Created Good*

Thus far, we have examined the biblical reasons for the occurrence of illness. We have yet to consider whether Scripture provide us with guidelines for evaluating the theological legitimacy of a medical tradition. To address this, we must answer a more fundamental question: "Why did God create humanity?" Genesis 1 answers this plainly: It is for humankind to enjoy God's love and His creation, as we live out our lives as stewards of His land. This is why Genesis calls the idyllic state when Creator, humanity and creation are in fellowship with each other, "very good" (Gen 1:31).

### *Our Fall did not Affect the Nature of Creation*

Unfortunately, our first ancestors disobeyed God and were banished from Paradise. Consequently, our relationship with God and His creation was fractured permanently. This being said, neither our sin nor Satan could damage the goodness of God's creation. It is not within our power to change the nature of creation. Paul makes this clear in 1 Timothy 4:3–5, when he declares that,

> *... everything God created is good, and nothing is to be rejected if it is received with thanksgiving, because it is consecrated by the word of God and prayer.*

Elsewhere in 1 Corinthians 8, Paul speaks of idols as nothing (1 Cor 8:4) and thus they have no power or influence over the nature of food. It is for this reason that Christians can partake in food sacrificed to idols. Indeed, "we are no worse if we do not eat, and no better if we do" (1 Cor 8:8). The only occasions we should not eat food offered to idols is when our actions stumble a weaker brother (1 Cor 8:7) or when the feasting is part of a religious ritual (1 Cor 10:14–16). In other words, when our partaking of the food is understood as participation in religious worship!

Putting these together, it is evident that the non-Christian or religious ideals imposed on any kind of food, or for that matter, any creature of God, does not alter their nature. A good case in point is the popular Chinese green tea, *Tie Guanyin*, or Iron Goddess of Mercy. Its Buddhist-sounding name does not, in any way, change its properties or nutritional value as green tea.

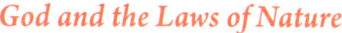

### *God and the Laws of Nature*

Besides this, it is important to remember that the God we worship is not a God of chaos but the God of order. The God who provides laws for His people. The corollary here is that the nature He created must likewise be invested with and governed by unchanging laws — the laws of nature. This was the premise that catalysed the modern scientific revolution and inspired numerous scientists from the seventeenth to nineteenth century to investigate the laws of nature, and articulate it through the use of mathematics. The most well-known, of course, are Newton's laws of classical mechanics.

Central to the modern scientific revolution is also the belief that these laws of nature can be discovered through the use of experimentation or empirical studies. This is true not only for modern physics and biology, but also medicine. This is why, from the late nineteenth century onwards, modern medicine has largely adopted experimentation, or double-blinded random controlled trials in particular, as the means for diagnosing diseases and assessing the efficacy of medical therapies.

### *Towards a Theology of Medicine*

What does this mean for our study of Western and Chinese medical traditions?

1. We need to recognise that the psychosomatic nature of human beings has not been changed by the Fall; it remains consistent irrespective of medical traditions. This "law of nature," readers must recognise, should also be differentiated from the medical theories known to our physicians, whether modern or Chinese. This is because the "law of nature" is the absolute truth of how our body operates, while our medical knowledge consists only of theories that we developed to describe the human body. Such theories are necessarily constrained by the limits of our human efforts.[5]

To put it differently, any form of medical therapy whether Chinese, modern or Indian, would have to adhere by the biological laws that God has invested in our human nature. Consequently, even when a medical theory does not provide an adequate explanation of aetiology (how diseases occur) or human physiology, its therapy can still be effective if it adheres to the laws of nature invested in the human being. On the other hand, even when a medical tradition can describe the human physiology more accurately, its therapy may not work if it does not adhere to the actual laws of our biological nature.

2. Since all medical therapies must comply with the laws of nature invested in our human bodies, their efficacies should be measurable by means of experiments or empirical studies. This is not to say, however, that we must rely solely on double-blinded random controlled trials, though this is often understood to be the case in the practice of modern medicine.

    A medical therapy is theologically legitimate if it can be tested empirically for its efficacy, since this provides evidence for the extent to which it is adhering by the laws of nature God has invested in human nature.

3. By extension, we can conclude that any form of therapy that cannot be assessed by empirical studies is illegitimate. Here, we mean explicitly religious forms of healing, such as the drinking of water mixed with burnt talisman, the calling of a deity to heal a patient or the use of particular qigong practices that call for spiritual aid in its therapy.[6]

EVALUATING
WESTERN
MEDICAL
TRADITIONS

# The Greek Origins of Western Medicine

## *Galenic-Hippocratic Medicine*

Now that we have worked out the theological principles for evaluating a medical tradition, we shall bring these to bear on both the Western and Chinese medical traditions. We begin with Western medical traditions, which include both Greek and modern medicine.

The early Christians, as mentioned earlier, largely employed the Galenic-Hippocratic medicine used by their Christian and non-Christian peers. Hippocratic medicine dates back to the fifth and fourth centuries BC, and initially comprised of diverse medical theories taught in a collection called the Hippocratic corpus. Then in second century AD, the famous physician Galen of Pergamum emphasised the doctrine of humours taught in particular Hippocratic texts. By the fourth century, this Galenic interpretation of Hippocratic medicine began to hold sway and would remain dominant right until the early nineteenth century.

What is the doctrine of humours? The doctrine begins with the premise that all things, or the stuff of creation, are made up of four basic elements: air, water, fire and earth. These elements, in turn, combine to form four types of humours: blood, phlegm, black bile and yellow bile. Different combinations of these humours then give us the different organs in the human body.

Sicknesses thus occur whenever the proportion of humours in our bodies goes awry. When this happens, one can treat the patient using drugs, massages, baths, surgery or cautery.

## *A 'Dot' Perspective of the World*

At this point, we may ask, what is the underlying assumption of this humoral theory? Basically this: We can only understand the world by breaking it down to its smallest building blocks or constituent parts and studying these elements. Once we grasp these elements, we should be able to work backwards and understand the more complex creations that they form. I coined this approach the 'Dot Perspective' of the world. It remains true even when Greek medicine eventually gave way to modern medicine.

## *Modern Medicine*

Galenic-Hippocratic medicine was abandoned in favour of modern biomedicine in the late nineteenth century. Since then, the causes of diseases have changed from humoral imbalances to bacteria, viruses, cancerous cells, genetic disorders or organ failures.

On the surface, it would seem that modern medicine differs significantly from Hippocratic medicine. This is true, and its new modern perspectives have certainly resulted in much medical and therapeutic breakthroughs. Having said that, both Greek and modern medicine still share the same philosophical premise: that the truth is to be grasped by understanding the smallest elements constituting the world or the human body.

This time round, it is no longer the humours but DNA, cells or organs that form the human body, or the bacteria and viruses that threaten it. They are different kinds of dots, but still a 'Dot Perspective' nevertheless.

## Reflections on the Dot Perspective of the World

### *Strengths*

Having examined the philosophical basis of Greek and modern medicine, we can now ask, "Are these medical theories and the Dot Perspective they assume theologically legitimate?"

The plain answer is that the Bible has *nothing* to say about the legitimacy of these medical theories. It is also silent about this dot or 'divide-and-conquer' approach to understanding the world. Simply said, such a philosophical premise is just a way by which limited human beings have learnt to cope with the complex realities of the world. This 'Dot Perspective' of the world has achieved much in the modern scientific revolution and transformed the world remarkably as we know it.

## *Weaknesses*

Having said that, this fragmentary approach to creation and its natures also assumes that there are no systemic relationships between the dots that we study. This, however, is not the case.

The sum of the dots is greater than the dots themselves. In other words, there is systemic information embedded in the relationships between the dots. When we deconstruct the nature of something down to its smallest elements, we inadvertently lose the systemic information holding the different dots together.

A good example of this is the supply chain of a television. While one can reduce costs or improve efficiencies of the supply chain by simply focusing on one node, such as the manufacturing plant or the warehouse, these productivity programmes may wreak havoc in other parts of the chain and lead to a deterioration of its performance and higher costs in the overall supply chain.[7]

## Limitations

Besides this, we must recognise that any form of medicine, modern medicine included, remains a product of our finite human effort. The knowledge we derive from our scientific research will therefore be limited. There will be blind spots, gaps and uncertainties in our knowledge. This is a sobering reality we must accept. As the Harvard physician and author Atu Gawande puts it,

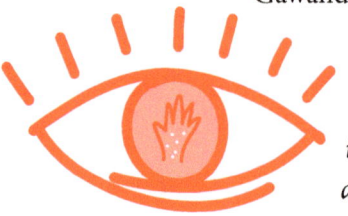

*... the story of medicine is the story of how we deal with the incompleteness of our knowledge and the fallibility of our skills.*[8]

EVALUATING
CHINESE
MEDICAL
TRADITIONS

# Introducing Chinese Philosophical Metaphors

We turn now to the Chinese medical tradition. As we shall see, since the beginning of Chinese philosophy, the Chinese never sought to understand the world by breaking it down to its constituent parts or elements. Instead, Chinese culture, including Chinese medicine, has generally emphasised the learning and understanding of how the different parts or 'dots' relate to one another. In other words, a systemic understanding of the world. Indeed, as early as the Han Dynasty (around 200 BC), Han Confucian philosophers already taught the concept of Heaven and Humanity Living in Unity: 天人合一 (*tianren heyi*). What is this heavenly unity? It is an aspiration for human beings to live in harmony (和 *he*) with the Heavens (or God) and the Earth (Creation). It is an idyllic state where the three are not opposed to but complement one another. How did the ancient Chinese express such harmonious relations? Well, through the concepts or metaphors of *yinyang* (阴阳), *qi* (气) and *wuxing* (五行). What are these metaphors? Are they religious or irreligious to begin with?

## *Yinyang*

We begin with the idea of *yinyang*. In Chinese philosophy, *yin* denotes attributes such as stillness, coldness, softness and femininity; while *yang* describes the opposite attributes like movement, hotness, hardness and masculinity. Both *yin* and *yang* do not exist independently or on their own. They always co-exist in mutually dependent relationships, where *yin* needs *yang* as much as *yang* needs *yin*. More importantly both *yin* and *yang* do not denote any specific natures or things. Rather, they are relational categories used for the description of relationships between any two entities.

Thus, A may be *yin* and B, *yang*, because A is softer than B. Yet, B can also be *yin* to C, if C is harder than B and so on. This concept of relationality is well illustrated in how Chinese medicine describes the relationships between different parts of the body.

- The back of a human body faces the sun and is thus regarded as *yang*. The front receives less sunlight and is thus denoted as *yin*. This being said, the upper part of the human torso, the chest area, is regarded as *yang* when compared to the lower part of the torso (the tummy area), which is *yin*.

- Likewise, the back of the palm faces the sun more and is thus regarded as *yang*, while the palm is *yin*.

By now, it should be clear that the idea of *yinyang* has nothing to do with the philosophy of nature, or as Western philosophers call it, ontology. There is nothing which is absolutely *yin* or *yang* by nature. A failure to grasp this difference has often misled theologians to regard *yinyang* as a form of Chinese or religious dualism. This is not the case at all.

## *Qi*

If *yinyang* denotes a mutuality and dependence between two entities, what then is the idea of *qi*? The traditional Chinese character of *qi* is 氣, which has the Chinese character of 米 or rice written within it. Basically, the earliest idea of *qi* has to do with the steam swirling over a hot bowl of rice. In other words, intrinsic to the idea of *qi* is swirling or flowing. When applied to Chinese medicine, *qi* essentially denotes the extent to which the flow of blood (气血 *qixue*) is regular, smooth or sufficient. When the flow is optimal, a human being is healthy. If the flow is insufficient (气虚 *qixu*), blocked (气阻 *qizu*) or flowing in the opposite/ wrong direction (逆气 *niqi*), illnesses occur. When an organ, such as the kidney, is described as weak (肾虚 *shenxu*), it is implied that the systemic flow of blood and nutrients in the kidney is inadequate, resulting in weaknesses and diseases in the kidney. The flow of *qi* in, to and from the kidney must then be altered to improve the organ's condition.

## *Wuxing*

If *yinyang* denotes the mutual dependence between two entities and *qi* the way or how they relate or influence each other, what then is the role of *wuxing* as a metaphor? *Wuxing* (五行) is sometimes called the five phases. They are metal, wood, water, fire and earth. On first glance, this looks similar to the Greek theory of the four elements. The only difference appears to be an additional element in the Chinese version. In actual fact, the two systems are very different. What is important in *wuxing* is not the nature or attribute of each *xing*/phase but the relation between a pair of phases.

For example, fire burns the earth and improves it by making it more fertile. Fire is thus seen as complementing earth. The two are mutually complementing or generating (相生 *xiangsheng*). On the other hand, water extinguishes fire and is thus opposed to fire. The two are mutually opposing or overcoming (相克 *xiangke*). Together, these five phases denote a system of relations where a phase opposes another phase while complementing a third:

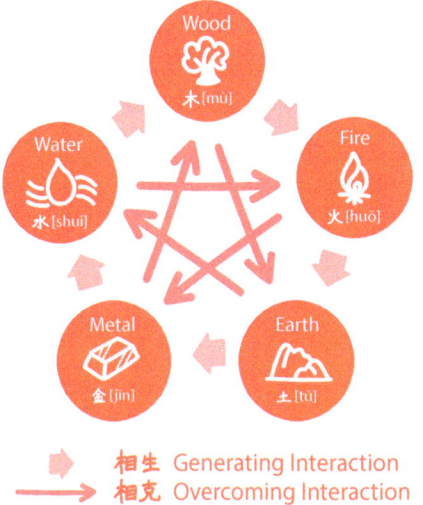

They then allow one to articulate the complex and intricate relationships between different entities or dots within a system, such as human physiology. For example, when applied in Chinese medicine, fire represents the heart while earth represents the spleen or indeed the digestive system. When the heart (fire) is strong, it is beneficial for the spleen/digestive system (earth). On the other hand, water represents the kidney and water can extinguish the fire (hurt the heart). In an ideal situation, the heart-fire and kidney-water should coordinate their flows to and through each other well. When an imbalance happens, the two start to threaten one another. This results in all sorts of illnesses, including chronic fatigue.

### *A Systemic View of Reality*

To summarise then, the metaphors of *yinyang*, *qi* and *wuxing* are regularly used in Chinese philosophy and medicine to articulate the intricate relationships in the world, be it between organs in the human bodies, relationships between human beings or those between different entities in the world. *Yinyang* enables one to describe the intimate relationship and dependence between two entities, while *qi* describes how one entity can affect or influence another. It also allows one to articulate the extent to which two entities' relationships are healthy or poor. Finally, *wuxing* enables us to describe their relationships further by denoting how an entity subsists in different relations with one another, sometimes opposing one entity while, at other times, complementing another.

## Chinese Metaphors and Medical History

When were these metaphors incorporated into Chinese medical discourse? To begin, we should note that many Chinese medical therapies, including acupuncture and moxibustion, were already in use before the Han Dynasty. The Han era, however, saw the introduction of these relational metaphors into Chinese medical theory. Henceforth, Han physicians would employ them in their aetiological and therapeutic discourse. This modelling language, if you will, remains in use till this day.

In particular, the metaphors were used to describe how the human organs (五脏六腑 *wuzang liufu*) are linked with the 12 meridians (经络 *jingluo*) traversing the human body to form a complex physiological network. A person falls ill whenever this organ-meridian network experiences a *yinyang* imbalance, and recovers when this balance is re-established. During the Han era, this was achieved largely through the use of acupuncture and moxibustion. By the Song Dynasty, Song physicians had found a way to employ drug therapy for treating this organ-meridian network. This is known as the concept of channel tropism or *guijing* (归经).

The Song physicians identified specific drugs that were efficacious for treating particular meridians and their respective organs. This therapeutic approach remains in practice till this day. For example, almond (杏仁) and Chinese bellflower (桔梗) are most apt for treating the lung meridian and thus the lungs. They are commonly prescribed for coughs and chest stuffiness. On the other hand, cinnabar (朱砂) is efficacious for the heart meridian and best used for treating heart ailments.

## Evaluating Chinese Medicine

### *Evaluating the Relational View of Reality*

Having explored Chinese philosophical metaphors and how they were incorporated in Chinese medical discourse through history, we are now ready to evaluate the theological legitimacy of Chinese medicine.

In short, just as the Western emphasis on ontology, or the 'Dot Perspective' of reality, is neither affirmed nor rejected by biblical teachings, so also the Chinese's relational or systemic perspective of reality. The Bible has nothing to say as to whether *yinyang* is right or wrong. Just as it has nothing to say about the validity of classical or quantum mechanics, DNA or the many scientific discoveries we have made through the centuries.

This being said, the Chinese ideal of Heaven and Humanity in Unity (*tianren heyi*) does parallel the idyllic state described in Genesis 1 — a state where relations between God, humanity and all creation are harmonious. A state of being "very good." To this extent then, we can say that there is a parallel between the Genesis ideal and the Chinese aspiration of all things subsisting in harmonious relations.

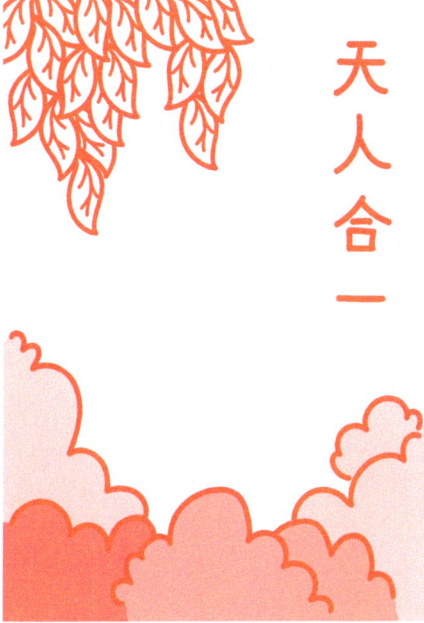

## The Empirical Basis of Chinese Medicine

Earlier, we mentioned that a medical theory or therapy is theologically legitimate only when it can be assessed empirically. This is because such validity implies that the theory or therapy is abiding, to some extent, to the laws of nature that God has invested in human nature.

With regards to empirical studies of Chinese therapy, it is clear that many Chinese therapies have not been validated by double-blinded random controlled clinical trials. The reason is simple; these therapies were invented way before the 1960s, when modern clinical trials became popular.

Nevertheless, this does not mean that Chinese therapies have not been validated empirically. Rather they have been tested through centuries of continual usage, where ineffective therapies or drug formulas were rejected, while useful ones were recorded and passed down through the medical classics and case records. The *Cold Damage Disorder Treatise* (伤寒杂病论 *shanghan zabinglun*) of the Han physician, Zhang Zhong Jing (张仲景) is a good case in point.

Zhang lived during the late Han era, when epidemics were rampant. Out of his 200 or so family members, almost two thirds died from epidemics, particularly Cold Damage disorders (伤寒 *shanghan*). Afflicted by such losses, Zhang vowed to treat such illnesses. After years of experiments and practice, he compiled his experience into the *Cold Damage Disorder Treatise*.

A thousand years later, during the Song era, the imperial library collected medical treatises from all over the country. This coincided with the breakout of epidemics in the country. It was not long before the newly discovered *Cold Damage Disorder Treatise* was consulted to treat these epidemics and its therapies were found to be useful. Henceforth the treatise was recognised as one of the key classics of Chinese medicine, and this has remained the case till this day. Zhang also became renowned as one of the greatest physicians in Chinese medical history.

Thus, while many Chinese medical therapies have not been subjected to the validation of modern-day clinical trials, they have gone through their own form of empirical validation. Or, as a physician friend of mine puts it, Chinese medical therapies have been subjected to centuries of clinical trials.

### *Limits of Chinese Medicine*

Despite its rich medical legacy, Chinese medicine, as a product of human invention, has its limitations.

1. It is unable to treat genetic disorders.

2. Its description of human physiology does not always cohere with that depicted in modern medicine. The Chinese understanding of the function of the spleen is a good example. In modern medicine, the spleen is responsible primarily for the production and removal of blood cells, and forms part of the immune system. In Chinese medical theory, however, the spleen is closely associated with the stomach. Both are taken jointly as representing the digestive system. Diseases of the spleen are thus digestive illnesses.

3. With Chinese medicine's encounter and dialogue with modern medical and technological developments, there is surely room for improvement. It is already happening in some areas: Laser technology is employed in acupuncture, robotics in massage and infra-red imaging in diagnosing meridians. And there is an opportunity for Chinese medical therapies to be further validated through the use of modern clinical trials.

# CONCLUSION

To conclude then, medicine is necessary because of the Fall, which led to the suffering, illness and death of all humankind. While the primal Fall is the primary cause of human illnesses, there are also secondary causes, ranging from divine punishment and spiritual training to illness being a religious symbol.

While the Scripture does not prescribe specific medical theories, it does provide a basis for evaluating the theological legitimacy of a medical discipline. Specifically, any medical therapy must adhere to the laws of nature invested in the human nature created by God. Its treatment is effective to the extent to which a therapy coheres with these laws. If it does not, the therapy fails, the patient's condition worsens, or he might even die. As to how one can decide the efficacy of such therapies, or if they abide by the laws of nature, this is best done through the use of empirical studies or experimentation.

As we have seen, both modern and Chinese medicine have adopted different approaches to developing their medical knowledge. One by adopting a 'Dot Perspective' of reality, while the other employs a systemic or relational approach. Both have also employed experimentation as a means of assessing the efficacy of their treatments. Both have yielded positive therapeutic results. Consequently, one might say that both medical traditions are theologically legitimate.

This being said, both, as human products, are also limited and are works in progress. There will always be room for improvement. Most importantly, we should realise that whether it is Chinese or modern medicine, both are means by which God heals us.

Ultimately, the true Healer of our illnesses remains Jesus Christ our Lord. No matter how we are healed, we would do well to ascribe glory to Him!

# Endnotes

1. "Acupuncture and Moxibustion of Traditional Chinese Medicine - Intangible Heritage - Culture Sector - UNESCO", accessed November 29, 2019, https://ich.unesco.org/en/RL/acupuncture-and-moxibustion-of-traditional-chinese-medicine-00425.
2. Daniel Tong, *A Biblical Approach to Chinese Tradition and Beliefs* (Singapore: Genesis, 2003), 108–24.
3. "TCM Service", *Bethel Community Services*, accessed January 4, 2016, http://www.bethelcs.org.sg/services/tcm-service/.
4. Jean-Claude Larchet, *The Theology of Illness* (Crestwood, N.Y.: St. Valdimir's Seminary Press, 2002), 26–33.
5. Such an approach to science is known as the philosophy of critical realism. It is the recognition that the reality we describe is not the true and absolute reality/laws of nature that exist. We do hope, however, that with more scientific investigation, we will be able to approach or better describe this absolute reality as clearly as possible.
6. For example, a qigong practitioner in China may be able to heal someone in Singapore by activating his *qi* in the spiritual realm. While the healing may be instantaneous, it is clearly healing by aid of a deity rather than abiding by the laws of human nature.
7. For example, to cope with excess television spare parts, a warehouse manager may build another warehouse to better manage the spare parts. This, however, will increase costs in the long run. A better approach would be to examine the costs of the entire supply chain, say by reducing the warranty period promised to customers. Fewer warranties to support will mean fewer spare parts and, therefore, lower costs.
8. "Why Doctors Fail", Atul Gawande, *The Guardian*, accessed October 1, 2019, https://www.theguardian.com/news/2014/dec/02/-sp-why-doctors-fail-reith-lecture-atul-gawande.

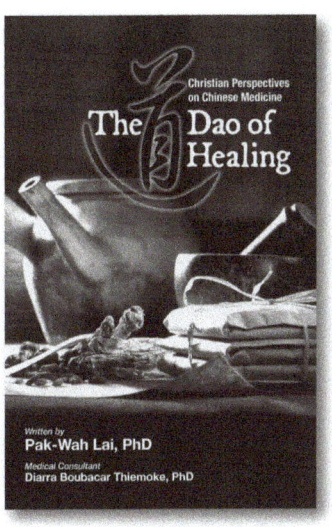

If you would like to learn more, read Dr Lai Pak-Wah's book, *The Dao of Healing: Christian Perspectives on Chinese Medicine*.

Paperback and eBook available at *graceworks.com.sg/store* and major online book retailers.

# GRACEW✦RKS

Graceworks is a publishing and training consultancy based in Singapore, dedicated to promoting spiritual friendship in church and society, and seeing lives transformed through books that present truth for life.

Our publications can be found on our online store, *www.graceworks.com.sg/store*. Our paperbacks and eBooks are also available at major online book retailers.

You can contact us at enquiries@graceworks.com.sg, or follow us on Facebook (@GraceworksSG) and Instagram (@graceworkssg).

www.ingramcontent.com/pod-product-compliance
Lightning Source LLC
LaVergne TN
LVHW051041070526
838201LV00067B/4882